The Secret Benefits of
AROMATHERAPY

The Secret Benefits of
AROMATHERAPY

Sumeet Sharma

Sterling Paperbacks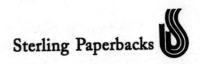

STERLING PAPERBACKS
An imprint of
Sterling Publishers (P) Ltd.
A-59, Okhla Industrial Area, Phase-II,
New Delhi-110020.
Tel: 26387070, 26386209; Fax: 91-11-26383788
E-mail: mail@sterlingpublishers.com
www.sterlingpublishers.com

The Secret Benefits of Aromatherapy
© 2008, Sterling Publishers Pvt. Ltd., New Delhi
ISBN 978 81 207 3996 3
Reprint 2011

Printed in India

Printed and Published by Sterling Publishers Pvt. Ltd.,
New Delhi-110 020.

Contents

Introduction

The word aromatherapy means 'treatment using scents'. It refers to the use of essential oils in Holistic Healing to improve health and emotional well-being and in restoring balance to the body. Essential oils are aromatic essences extracted from plants, flowers, trees, fruit, bark, grasses and seeds. There are more than 150 types of oils that can be extracted. These oils have distinctive therapeutic, psychological and physiological properties that improve health and prevent illness. All essential oils have unique healing and valuable antiseptic properties. Some oils are anti-viral, anti-inflammatory, pain-relieving, anti-depressant, stimulating, relaxing, expectorating, support digestion and have diuretic properties too.

Essential oils get absorbed into our body and exert an influence on it. The residue gets dispersed from the body naturally. They can also affect our mind and emotions. They enter the body in three ways: by inhalation, absorption and consumption.

From the chemist's point of view, essential oils are a mixture of organic compounds viz., ketones, terpenes, esters, alcohol, aldehyde and hundreds of other molecules which are extremely difficult to classify, as they are small and complex. The essential oils' molecules are small. They penetrate human skin easily and enter the blood stream directly and finally get flushed out through our elementary system.

A concentrate of essential oils is not greasy; it is more like water in texture and evaporates quickly. Some of them are light liquid insoluble in water and evaporate instantly when exposed to air. It would take 100 kg. of lavender to yield three kg. of lavender oil; one would need eight million jasmine flowers to yield barely one kg. of jasmine oil.

Some of these aroma oils are very expensive. They are extracted using maceration. The purification process called defleurage is employed, and in some cases fat is used instead of oil. Then this process, called enfleurage, is used for final purification.

Some of the common essential oils used in aromatherapy for their versatile application are:
- Clary Sage (Salvia Scarea)
- Eucalyptus (Eucalyptus Globulus)
- Geranium (Pelargonium Graveolens)
- Lavender (Lavendula Vera Officinals)

- Lemon (Citrus Limonem)
- Peppermint (Mentha Piperita)
- Petitgrain (Citus Aurantium Leaves)
- Rosemary (Rosmarinus Officinals)
- Tea-tree (Melaleuca Alternifolia)
- Ylang Ylang (Cananga Odorata)

The oils mentioned can be included in a beginners kit.

Origin of Aromatherapy

The oldest use of aroma oils is known to be as old as 6000 years back when Egyptian physician, Imhotep, the then God of Medicine and Healing recommended fragrant oils for bathing and massaging. In 4,500 B.C. Egyptians used myrrh and cedarwood oils for embalming their dead and 6,500 years later the preserved mummies prove the fact discovered by the modern researchers that the cedarwood contains natural fixative and strong antibacterial and antiseptic properties.

Hippocrates, the Greek father of medicine, recommended regular aromatherapy baths and scented massages. This is what he effectively used to ward off plague from Athens.

Romans utilised essential oils for pleasure and to cure pain and also for their popular perfumed baths and massages. Emperor Nero being indulgent in orgies, feasts and fragrances employed rose oil frequently to cure his headaches, indigestion and to maintain his high spirits while enjoying amusements.

During the great plague in London in 1665, people burnt bundles of lavender, cedarwood and cypress in the streets and carried posies of the same plants as their only defence to combat infectious diseases.

Aromatherapy received a wider acceptance in the early twentieth century. In 1930s Rene-Maurice-Gatte Fosse, a French chemist, dipped his burnt hand in lavender oil. To his surprise the wound healed very quickly without any infection or scarring. He did considerable research on various oils and their therapeutic and psychotherapeutic properties.

Dr Jean Volnet, French army surgeon extensively used essential oils in World War II. It was Madame Morquerite Murry who gave the holistic approach to aroma oils by experimenting with them for individual problems.

Today, research has proved the multiple use of aroma oils. Medical research in the recent years has uncovered the fact that the odours we smell have a significant impact on the way we feel. Smells act directly on the brain like a drug according to scientific research. For instance smelling lavender increases alpha wave frequency in the back of the head and this state is associated with relaxation.

Essential oils, like spiritual healing (Reiki, Pranic, Magnetic), homeopathic, herbal and flower remedies have a life force that vibrates within the body and the benefit exerted is too subtle to evaluate.

How Do Aroma Oils Work?

Dr Alan Huch, a neurologist, psychiatrist and also the director of Smell and Taste Research Centre in Chicago says, "Smell acts directly on the brain, like a drug." Our nose has the capacity to distinguish 1,00,000 different smells, (many of which) affect us without our knowing about it.

The aroma enters our nose and comes in contact with the cilia, the fine hair inside the nose lining. The receptors in the cilia are linked to the olfactory bulb which is at the end of the smell tract. The end of the tract is in turn connected to the brain itself. Smells are converted by cilia into electrical impulses that are transmitted to the brain through olfactory system. All the impulses reach the limbic system. Limbic system is that part of the brain which is associated with our moods, emotions, memory and learning. All the smell that reaches the limbic system has a direct chemical effect on our moods.

For example smelling lavender increases alpha waves in the brain and it is this wave that helps us to relax. A whiff of jasmine increases beta waves in the brain and this wave is associated with an increased agile and alert state.

Limbic system is also a storehouse of millions of remembered smells. That is why the mere fragrance of haystack takes us back to childhood.

The molecular size of the essential oils is very tiny and they can easily penetrate through the skin and get into the blood stream. It takes anything between a few seconds to two hours for the essential oils to enter the skin and within four hours the toxins get out of the body through urine, perspiration and excreta.

Aroma oils work like magic for stress-related problems, psychosomatic disorders, skin infections, hair loss, inflammations, pains arising from muscular or skeletal disorders to name some. Actually essential oils have innumerable applications.

In Bristol, lavender oil was used on 28 patients who had undergone bypass surgery. 24 of them reported reduced breathing rates, lower blood pressure and anxiety levels.

In Paris, in 1985, 28 women were given treatment for thrush using essential oils. After 90 days the clinical examination showed that 21 of them had been cured completely.

Essential oils are safe to use. The only caution being they should never be used directly because some oils may irritate sensitive skin or cause photosensitivity. They should be blended in adequate proportion with the carrier oils. A patch test is necessary to rule out any reactions.

Various Uses of Aroma Oils

Essential oils can be used in a variety of ways at home and place of work. Some of the common ways are:

Inhalation: Add 2-3 drops of essential oil depending on which oil you have selected to the hot boiling water and inhale the steam by covering your head with a towel to stop the steam from escaping. Steaming also helps open the pores of the skin and thus more oil is absorbed giving the additional benefit of a facial. The bowl which has hot water and the aroma oil could be left under the bed so that the room is enveloped in aromatic fragrance. This could be done with the same bowl of hot steaming water and essential oil which had been used earlier for inhalation. A drop or two sprinkled on a handkerchief can give a lasting benefit of the aroma oil. For a very peaceful and relaxed sleep one or two drops of essential oils on a tissue kept inside the pillow or cushion could be used.

Diffusers and Vaporisers: Diffusers are generally made of ceramic or clay. The diffuser has a cave-like opening to house small candles or earthen oil lamps and the top is shaped like a curved cup to hold a little water and few drops of aroma oil. Fill the top cup with water, add a few drops of essential oils depending on the oil chosen then light the candle or the lamp. For the oil lamp to last for a long duration, add castor oil to the earthen lamp because castor oil burns for a very long time as compared to the other oils used to light a lamp. Once the water and oil heat up, evaporation takes place and the whole atmosphere is filled with the aromatic scent. The process of evaporation continues for nearly five to six hours. This is ideal for presenting a conducive ambience during a gathering or even in bedrooms, hotels, living-rooms, etc., or any place where scented air is required. One can get instant relief from pain, a relaxed and positive feeling prevails when the right oil is used. One needs to be careful in choosing the right essential oil.

Vaporisers are normally used as insect repellents in the form of mats or other types of vaporisers. One could reuse the used mats by adding 2-3 drops of essential oil of your own choice and keeping them lit (electrically). Slowly, the smell will get released and the area would be filled with soothing aroma. Lemon or rosemary are beneficial for offices, lavender for bedroom, antiseptic tea-tree for disinfecting a sick room and citronella for repelling the insects.

Massage: The most common form of treatment is massage because the dual benefits of touch therapy and scent therapy are simultaneously enjoyed. Massage improves the circulation of the blood, tones the muscles, detoxifies the body, releases trapped energy from tense muscles. The fragrance triggers a sense of pleasure and well-being. The penetration of essential oil through the skin during massages is high. Generally carrier oils like sunflower, coconut, olive, sweet almond, sesame and vegetable oils are mixed with aroma oils. The aroma oils should not be used for massages directly without dilution. About 10 drops or 1 teaspoon of essential oil can be mixed to about 30 ml of carrier oil. This makes a very rejuvenating massage oil.

Baths: This is an easy way to relax using essential oils. Add the selected oil to your bathtub, stir the water well and spend 20 minutes in the tub. The aroma oil enters the body through the skin to give lasting benefits. Just a few drops are required to be added to the bathtub. The essential oils can also be added to a bucket of water instead of a bathtub. Mix the oil in the water properly, as some of the aroma oils are insoluble in water.

Foot Bath: You can immerse your feet in a bowl of lukewarm water to which 2-3 drops of essential oil is added. This is a very refreshing experience after a hard days work and if you have sweaty and smelly feet then too this foot bath is very beneficial.

Potpourri: Potpourri as the name suggests is a mixture of dried flowers, herbs, grass and seed pods. Few drops of essential oil added to the potpourri and kept in a bowl would keep giving out aromatic fragrance for 4-6 weeks. Another more effective method would be to keep the potpourri mixture after adding the essential oil in a closed container overnight so that the oil gets absorbed. The following morning the box can be kept open and the lingering aroma would fill the area.

Bedtime: Sprinkle 2-3 drops on the pillow cover or on a tissue that can be placed under the pillow or cushion cover and inhaled just before sleeping or while sleeping. This can be very useful in treating headaches, stress, tension and in boosting confidence. Some of the essential oils act as an aphrodisiac too.

Compresses: Both cold and hot compresses are good for health. Add 2-3 drops of aroma oil to a bowl of hot (depending on how much of heat you can withstand) or warm water and dip a hand towel or piece of cotton to enable it to absorb the mixture then squeeze out the excess water and place the towel or cotton on the area to be treated. Leaving the compress on the area for two hours is quite beneficial. Oil like lavender is usually used. This provides relief when used over bruises, skin problems and premenstrual syndromes. To make cold compress, add 6 cubes of ice to a bowl with 2-3 drops of essential oil and dip a hand towel or a piece of cotton to absorb the mixture then squeeze out the excess water and place the towel or cotton on the area to be treated. Cold compress is highly helpful in treating burns, sore feet, hangover, sprains and headaches. After a facial the use of hot and cold compress, alternately, helps the skin.

Oral Intake: It is an accepted practice abroad to take essential oil orally as it is safe. However, care should be taken only under the supervision or guidance of an experienced aromatherapy practitioner. Few oils can be taken internally in a prescribed dosage for a particular problem like indigestion only under the guidance of a qualified therapist.

Beauty Treatment: Aroma oils have been used as an application for the skin from times immemorial. As they are highly soothing in treating and enhancing the natural beauty of the skin they can be safely incorporated in facials, massages, manicures, pedicures, scalp treatment, hair wash, hair treatment along with other creams and oils. Rose, chamomile, lemon, lavender, geranium, sandalwood are some good oils for general use for facials irrespective of the fact that beauty treatment is given to normal, mature, dry, oily, sensitive or problem skin. Either one of these or a combination of two of them could be used. The carrier oils that are helpful in a beauty treatment are sweet almond, wheat germ, peach kernel, apricot kernel and sunflower. Steam facials with essential oils are also rejuvenating and help in improving the skin texture.

Room Sprays: There is a call for protecting the environment and this is becoming a prime concern worldwide. Aerosols are being discouraged due to their ozone depleting properties. Essential oils are natural and hence they could be used liberally to deodorise a room, freshen and scent your bathroom, living-room, bedroom, dining-room, office cabin, etc. Merely add 10-12 drops of aroma oil to half a litre of water and spray the mixture with the help of a spray bottle. Oils like lavender, lemon, peppermint, pine and rosemary are best for this application. Cupboards, wardrobes can also be disinfected. If a room smells of dampness or there are moulds in the hotel rooms, houses, offices or factories and shops the essential oil along with water can be sprayed.

Insect Repellents: Essential oils are excellent fragrant dispenser and non toxic insecticides. Just 2-3 drops of essential oil can be used on pillow covers, mattresses or used mosquito mats (this can be electrically reused) or applied to the exposed skin after blending with carrier oil before going to bed. Lemongrass is best for flying insects, tea-tree for ants and fleas, thyme for crawling pests, camphor for moths and citronella for mosquitoes. Even delicate plants (both indoor and outdoor) can be protected from insects by spraying the above essential oils to the roots of the plant.

Miscellaneous Uses: Aroma oil can be added to the water used for cleaning the house. It can be used to wipe the kitchen counter, platform, dining tables, babies' nappies for disinfecting purpose and also to wash the baths and toilets.

Aroma oils have versatile applications and innumerable benefits and can be made a part of our daily routine.

Essential Oils and Their Benefits

Amrette Seed

Botanical name: Abelmoschus Moschatus
Plant part: Seeds
Properties: Warmth-giving, relaxing, stimulating, calming
Quantity: 2-3 drops
Application: Helpful in relieving anxiety, fatigue, depression or other stress-related conditions, muscular aches, pains, cramps and poor circulation. Is an aphrodisiac. Excellent to freshen up tired and hurting feet.
Precaution: Use in low dosage. Avoid very frequent massages or baths.

Aniseed

Botanical name: Pimpenella Anisum
Plant part: Seed pod
Properties: Warming, stimulating
Quantity: 3-5 drops

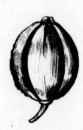

Application: Digestive stimulant. Helpful in treating coughs, bronchitis and catarrh.

Angelica

Botanical name: Angelica Archangelica
Plant part: Root, seed, fruit
Properties: Expectorant, digestive stimulant, relaxing
Quantity: 2-3 drops
Application: Useful for colds, coughs, flu, muscular pains and aches, rheumatism. Helps in digestion. Also useful in healing smoker's cough.
Precaution: Avoid during pregnancy. Can cause photosensitivity so avoid exposure to sun after use.

Basil

Botanical name: Ocimum Basilicum
Part of Plant: Leaves
Properties: Uplifting, refreshing
Quantity: 2-3 drops
Application: Good for students and executives. Helps in relieving nervous tension, stress, mild anxiety, nausea, indigestion, flatulence, loss of appetite, temporarily relieves cough, sinusitis, flatulence, cold, fever, bronchitis, earaches, eases muscular pains, spasm, rheumatic and arthritic pains. It also acts as an insect repellent.
Precaution: Avoid during pregnancy.

Bergamot

Botanical name: Citrus Aurantium
Part of Plant: Peel of the fruit
Properties: Calming, refreshing, rejuvenating
Quantity: 3-5 drops
Application: Heals wounds and relieves ulcers, treats eczema, psoriasis (stress related) and PMT (Pre Menstrual Tension). Works as an appetiser. Beneficial in treating oily skin problems. Relieves respiratory infections viz. bronchitis, sore throat and tonsillitis, colic, flatulence and indigestion. Beneficial in treating anxiety, depression, mental and psychological disturbances. Acts as an antiseptic for urinary tract problem, cystitis. Effective in treating cold sores, chickenpox and shingles.
Precaution: Avoid using on sensitive skin as it can cause irritation. Avoid exposure to sun as it can increase skin's photosensitivity.

Black Pepper

Botanical name: Piper Nigrum
Plant Part: Berry
Properties: Warming, strengthening
Quantity: 2-3 drops
Application: Helps in relieving muscular aches, pains, stiffness, fatigue. Useful in relieving physical and emotional problems. Gives temporary relief from

arthritis, fibrosis, cold, flu, indigestion, respiratory infections, chills, catarrh. Helps in curing colic, flatulence, indigestion, heartburn and loss of appetite. Helps to maintain peripheral circulation, eases chilblains and tones muscles. Increases concentration and alertness.

Precaution: Use in moderation.

Camphor

Botanical name: Cinnamomum Camphora
Plant part: Wood
Properties: Relieving
Quantity: 2-3 drops
Application: Helps in treating coughs, colds, fevers, rheumatism, arthritis constipation, insomnia, sprains, depression, acne and inflamed skin.
Precaution: Use in moderation.

Cardamom

Botanical name: Elettaria Cardomumum
Plant part: Seeds
Properties: Warming
Quantity: 2-3 drops
Application: Helps in relieving nausea, coughs, headaches, aches, digestion and it is a tonic.
Precaution: Use in moderation.

Chamomile

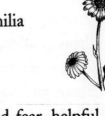

Botanical name: Matricaria Chamomilia
Plant part: Flowers
Properties: Soothes
Quantity: 3-5 drops
Application: Eases anxiety, anger and fear, helpful in treating insomnia, used for colitis, gastritis, diarrhoea, urinary tract infection, menopause and menstrual related problems. Relieves stress, depression and irritability related to PMT. Helps to relieve muscular pains, inflammation of arthritic joints and swollen joints. It is used in treating skin problems viz. psoriasis, dermatitis and eczema. Mild on children facing teething problem and earache. Soothes burns, blisters, inflamed wounds, broken capillaries. It can be used to lighten fair hair.
Precaution: Avoid during pregnancy.

Clove Bud

Botanical name: Syzygium Aromaticum
Plant part: Buds
Properties: Warming and soothing
Quantity: 1-2 drops
Application: Relieves aches and pains (joints). Rheumatoid sprains, asthma, colds, flu, colic, dyspepsia, nausea, diarrhoea, toothache, ulcers, wounds, bronchitis, nervous tension, depression and stress. It is

used as an effective antiseptic, and analgesic antibacterial. Useful as mosquito repellent and in fighting acne. Helps relieve athlete's foot and cuts.
Precaution: Use in low moderation. Avoid during pregnancy.

Cedarwood

Botanical name: Cedrus Deodora
Plant part: Wood shaving, sawdust
Properties: Sedating and relaxing
Quantity: 5-7 drops
Application: Helps relieve stress, tension, mild anxiety, arthritis, rheumatism, itching and dandruff. Symptoms of acne, pimple, oily skin, inflamed skin, eczema and blemishes can be temporarily relieved. Aids in clearing catarrh, congestion and sinusitis. Useful as insect repellent too.
Precaution: Avoid during pregnancy.

Cypress

Botanical name: Cupressus Sempervirens
Plant part: Needles, twigs
Properties: Refreshing, calming and strengthening
Quantity: 2 drops
Application: An astringent to circulation, haemorrhoids, varicose veins, cellulite; brings down external bleeding and excessive perspiration and heavy menstrual flow; useful in asthma, bronchitis, dry cough, cold and flu.

Helps to heal swollen breasts.

Precaution: Avoid during pregnancy.

Clary Sage

Botanical name: Salvia Sclarea

Plant part: Flowering tops

Properties: Euphoric, sensual, warming and relaxing

Quantity: 2-5 drops

Application: Useful in dealing with anxiety, stress, tension and migraine, menstrual cramps and pains, PMT, muscular tension, excessive perspiration. Is warming and relaxing. Brings down high blood pressure and excessive sebum. Reduces post natal depression and eases childbirth by encouraging labour. Immune system gets strengthened. Eases asthma.

Precaution: Can cause drowsiness, avoid when under alcoholic effect. Avoid during pregnancy and also if one suffers from epilepsy.

Eucalyptus

Botanical name: Eucalyptus Globulus

Plant part: Leaves, twigs

Properties: Cooling and clearing

Quantity: 2-3 drops

Application: Clears stuffed nose and head. Acts as a decongestant; cures fever, cold. Relieves stress, fatigue, muscular pains, sprains, aches, rheumatism, headaches, sinusitis and mild respiratory infections. It is

anti-inflammatory. Quite useful in treating wounds, burns, boils, abscesses, blisters, cold, shingles, blemishes, insect bites, anti-bacterial and is an insect repellent too.
Precaution: Can irritate skin. Keep away from children.

Fennel

Botanical name: Foeniculum Vulgare
Plant part: Seeds
Properties: Calming
Quantity: 2-3 drops
Application: Useful in easing colic, constipation and digestion problems, fluid retention, cellulite, menstrual pain, PMT, menopause, nausea, flatulence and loss of appetite. Helps in fighting hangovers, increases flow of breast milk and relieves bronchitis. Cures kidney stones and relieves intestinal spasm. Has a mild diuretic and laxative effect.
Precaution: Avoid during pregnancy.

Frankincense

Botanical name: Olibanum Boswellia Carterii
Plant part: Gum resin
Property: Fortifying, soothing
Quantity: 3-5 drops
Application: Helps in meditation; slows and deepens breathing. Fortifies emotionally against nightmares, fear and grief. Balances and opens Crown chakra. It helps in healing ulcers and infected wounds. Treats dry,

wrinkled, inflamed skin. It also cures coughs, laryngitis, asthma, catarrh and bronchitis. It reduces scar and promotes healing. Aids in maintaining supple skin by toning it.

Geranium

Botanical name: Pelargonium Graveolens
Plant part: Leaves, stalk, flower
Properties: Calming, balancing, relaxing, refreshing
Quantity: 5-7 drops
Application: Helps to deal with nervous tension, anxiety, mood swings, depression, menopause problems, hot flushes, post natal depression, PMT, irregular menstruation. Treats swollen and painful breasts, fluid retention problems, emotional outbursts, irritability, throat infections. It cures colds, flu, neuralgia, sciatica, acne, bruises, burns, cuts, dermatitis, eczema, mature skin and mouth ulcers. Normalises skin imbalances. Works as insect repellant, harmonises and calms. It also acts as an astringent and cleanser.

Ginger

Botanical name: Zingiber Officinale
Plant part: Root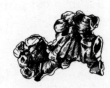
Properties: Warming, stimulating
Quantity: 2 drops

Application: Relieves colic, cramp, flatulence, nausea, travel sickness and indigestion. Cures migraine, coughs, congestion, common cold, catarrh, influenza, sore throat, sinusitis, arthritic pains, rheumatism, muscular aches, sprains and strains. Helps in blood circulation and aids memory. Heals bones and brings down temperature in fever also. Relieves morning sickness (if inhaled) in pregnancy and hangovers. Stimulates circulation, relaxes blood vessels and can also help ease angina.

Precaution: May irritate sensitive skin. Use in moderation.

Juniper Berry

Botanical name: Juniperus Communis
Plant part: Berries
Properties: Uplifting, refreshing, relaxing.
Quantity: 2-3 drops
Application: Used to relieve stress, anxiety, pains of joints and rheumatic pain. Heals bruises, cramps, acne, colic, coughs, arthritis, menstrual pain, less menstrual flow, swollen and painful breasts (premenstrual). Deals with fluid retention, cellulite, obesity, poor circulation, haemorrhoids, loss of appetite. Tones the skin.

Precaution: Avoid during pregnancy and if suffering from high blood pressure. Can irritate the kidneys if used in excess.

Lavender

Botanical name: Lavandula Angustifolia
Plant part: Flowers
Quantity: 5-10 drops
Properties: Harmonising, soothing, balancing, refreshing, relaxing, calming
Application: Aids in relieving irritability (in adults and children as well), anxiety, stress. Relieves muscular aches and pains, bites and stings. Cures colds, flu, insomnia, headache, minor burns and scalds. It is antifungal and antibacterial so it is very useful in treating wounds. It can be used directly to relieve pain of minor burns and scalds. It balances and harmonises the body.
Precaution: Avoid during early pregnancy.

Lemon

Botanical name: Citrus Limon
Plant part: Peel of the fruit
Properties: Rejuvenating, enlivening, cooling, uplifting
Quantity: 3-6 drops
Application: Helps in healing bronchial problems, colds, flu, fever, sore throat, mouth ulcers, hormonal headaches, poor circulation, high blood pressure, wounds, stress, nervous tension and counteracts acidity, aids in clearing freckles and to rid warts. Useful for students and executives. Helps in stopping hot flushes

in menopause. It has a refreshing aroma and is an effective insect repellent too.

Precaution: Causes photosensitivity on sensitive skin. Avoid using when going out in sun as it may irritate sensitive skin.

Lemon-grass

Botanical name: Cymbogen Citratus
Plant part: Grass
Properties: Tranquilizing, soothing calming, refreshing
Quantity: 1-3 drops
Application: Helps in relieving shock, grief, trauma, depression and stress. Helps to fight lethargy, irritability during PMT and menopause, insomnia, excitability in children, chronic diarrhoea triggered due to emotional reasons. Improves skin elasticity, thread veins, stretch marks and scars. It gives relief from headaches, sore throat and mild respiratory problems. Helps in opening the skin pores, treating oily skin, curing acne and relieves indigestion.
Precaution: Avoid during pregnancy. It can also irritate skin.

Marjoram

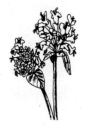

Botanical name: Origanum Marjorana
Plant part: Flowers, leaves
Properties: Calming, warming
Quantity: 3-5 drops

Application: Relieves anxiety, stress, high blood pressure, arthritis, rheumatism, swollen joints, asthma, colds, flu, sinusitis. Cures migraines, stomach and menstrual cramps, indigestion, constipation and flatulence. Calming to the nervous system. Reduces sexual urges, heals bruises.

Precaution: Use in moderation. Avoid during pregnancy.

Neroli

Botanical name: Citus Aurantium
Plant part: Petals
Properties: Calming, soothing, refreshing
Quantity: 1-3 drops
Application: Relieves mental lethargy, headaches, irritability caused due to menopause and PMT. It cures chronic diarrhoea due to emotional state and thread veins. Cures dryness, improves elasticity, sensitivity of skin and is also kind on mature skin. Calms excitable and restless children when used in baths before going to bed. Helps during shocks, trauma, grief and stress. Highly calming to those suffering from anxiety and fears. Helps lighten stretch marks and scars. Soothes palpitation, stress-related problems and depression. Helps during pregnancy and labour.

Orange (Sweet)

Botanical name: Citrus Aurantium
Plant part: Peel

Properties: Calming, refreshing
Quantity: 2-3 drops
Application: Effective in healing mouth ulcers, treats nervous tension, stress and anxiety. Gives relief from bronchial coughs, colds, flu and insomnia. Eases constipation and diarrhoea. It is very gentle on children brings down the fever.
Precaution: May increase skin photosensitivity. Avoid use before going out in the sun.

Palmarosa

Botanical name: Cymbopogon Martinii
Plant part: Grass
Properties: Clarifying, uplifting calming, refreshing
Quantity: 4-5 drops
Application: Stimulates cell regeneration, circulation, appetite. It maintains a supple skin, removes scars, helpful in treating acne, dermatitis balances sebum production, relieves indigestion, colds, flu, viruses and reduces fever.

Peppermint

Botanical name: Mentha Piperita
Plant part: Leaves
Properties: Cooling, invigorating comforting, refreshing, calming
Quantity: 1-3 drops

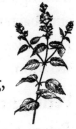

Application: A decongestant which gives relief from asthma, colds, flu, fever, headaches, toothaches, sinusitis, nausea, travel sickness, stomach upsets and indigestion, hangover. Cools skin inflammation, burns and sunburns as it is a very refreshing skin oil. Repels mosquitoes, mice and rats.

Precaution: Avoid during early pregnancy. Use in moderation as it can irritate sensitive skin.

Patchouli

Botanical name: Pogostemon Cabin
Plant part: Leaves
Properties: Exotic, calming, relaxing, enlivening, warming
Quantity: 2-4 drops
Application: Exotic aroma often used in perfumery. Emotionally enlivening, excites the senses. Helps in relieving anxiety, stress and depression. Helps to heal chapped rough skin, wounds and sores. Being anti-inflammatory it helps cool inflamed skin. Effective in treating dandruff, scars. It is an antiseptic, astringent, anti-bacterial and insect repellent.

Precaution: Use in moderation as excess dose can cause sedation.

Petitgrain

Botanical name: Citrus Aurantium var Amara
Plant part: Leaves

Properties: Clarifying, soothing, uplifting
Quantity: 4-5 drops
Application: Relieve mental strain, restlessness, anxiety, tension, stress, flatulence, dyspepsia and constipation. Helps in stimulating digestion and poor memory. Brings down acne. Reduces excessive perspiration, treats greasy skin and hair. Helps to build up immunity.

Pine

Botanical name: Pinus Sylvestris
Plant part: Needles
Properties: Invigorating, refreshing
Quantity: 1-3 drops
Application: Relieves muscular aches, pains, Arthritis, rheumatism, poor circulation, asthma, bronchitis, coughs, catarrh, sinusitis, sore throats, colds, flu, nervous exhaustion, stress, fatigue, neuralgia, sciatica and poor concentration. Heals cuts and abrasions, and reduces excessive perspiration. It is also an effective insect repellent.

Rose

Botanical name: Rose Centifoda damascena
Plant part: Flowers and leaves
Properties: Exciting, balancing
Quantity: 1-4 drops
Application: Helps to ease depression, frigidity, nervous tension, headache and insomnia. Relieves asthma,

shock, palpitations, poor circulation, dry coughs and nausea. Treats PMT, irregular or heavy menstruation, menstrual pain, impotence, irritability. Balances hormones. Useful also for dry, chapped, aging skin and eczema.

Rosemary

Botanical name: Rosemarinus officinalis
Plant part: Flowers, leaves
Properties: Reviving, invigorating, focusing, refreshing
Quantity: 2-4 drops
Application: Useful tonic for hair as it keeps dandruff at bay, clears lice, adds lustre to the hair. Useful in relieving stress, mental fatigue, anxiety, muscular aches and pains, rheumatism, arthritis, gout, sinusitis, migraine colds, flu, asthma, respiratory problem, poor circulation, fluid retention, cellulite, menstrual cramps, scanty flow during menstruation. Helps aid better concentration and clarity while studying.
Precaution: Avoid during pregnancy, if suffering from blood pressure or epilepsy.

Sandalwood

Botanical name: Santalum Album
Plant part: Wood
Properties: Strengthening, sedating, calming, relaxing
Quantity: 2-5 drops

Application: Helps to relieve nervous tension, depression, stress, anxiety, irritability, insomnia, dry coughs, sore throat, bronchitis, nausea, travel sickness. Heals inflamed, cracked, dry, chapped, aging skin, acne, blemishes and scars. Acts as a deodoriser in case of excessive perspiration. Excites the senses. It is an effective insect repellent.

Tarragon

Botanical name: Artemisia Dracunculus
Plant part: Leaves
Properties: Calming
Quantity: 2-3 drops
Application: Useful in relieving stomach disorders, nervousness leading to butterflies or knots in the stomach, indigestion, flatulence, PMT, cramps and constipation. It is antispasmodic, antiseptic and slightly diruretic
Precaution: Avoid during pregnancy. Use in moderation.

Tea-tree

Botanical name: Melaleuca Alternifolia
Plant part: Leaves, twigs
Properties: Soothing
Quantity: 2-5 drops
Application: Helpful in healing fungal and yeast infections, colds, influenza, cold sores, warts, burns,

shock, bacterial and viral infections, stings, herpes, nappy rash and hysteria.

Thyme (White)

Botanical name: Thymus Vulgaris
Plant part: Leaves, flowers
Properties: Stimulating, invigorating
Quantity: 2 drops
Application: Helpful in relieving tension, fatigue, anxiety, headaches, skin irritations, coughs, colds, rheumatic aches and pains. Useful insect repellent. It is a good stimulant and expectorant.
Precaution: Avoid during pregnancy. Use in moderation.

Vetiver

Botanical name: Vetiveria Zizanoides
Plant part: Roots
Properties: Balancing, calming, grounding
Quantity: 1-3 drops
Application: Helpful in relieving nervous tension, stress, muscular aches, pains, sprains, stiffness, arthritis, rheumatism, palpitation, congestion. Heals acne, blemishes, cuts and wound.

Ylang Ylang

Botanical name: Cananga Odorata
Plant part: Flowers

Properties: Balancing, relaxing

Quantity: 2-3 drops

Application: Helps to relieve tension, uncontrolled anger, stress, anxiety, rapid heart rate, rapid breathing, useful in high blood pressure, menopause, PMT, insomnia, impotence, frigidity, scalp conditioner. Useful in skin care.

Precaution: Avoid using after consuming alcohol or before driving. Use in moderation. It may cause headache and nausea when taken in excess.

How to Select Aroma Oils?

It is a fact that we get automatically attracted to pleasant smell and drift away from unpleasant smells. Subconsciously, we react to smells that fall in the range of these two extreme categories. The fragrance of freshly prepared food activates the saliva when one is hungry and newly cut grass relaxes a person who is highly stressed. Aromatherapy is based on this instinctive response to smell.

An alarm clock could be preset to release a particular scent you wish to wake up to. Patients could be made to relax by inhaling smell before undergoing a therapy. Automobile manufacturers could develop air conditioners with a preset mechanism to discharge aromas to keep the drivers alert while driving.

There are two simple tests to train your nose to learn and memorise the various smells. Test I would tell you how good your sense of smell is and Test II would tell you which aroma or essential oil you like the best.

Test I: Sniff and Tell Test

Blindfold your eyes and ask your friend or a family member to bring ten items from your kitchen . Let your partner allow you to sniff the item one by one and then try to recognise them by their aroma without actually seeing them. The items could be freshly cut citrus fruit, freshly crushed herbs, jars containing pickle, sauce etc. Place the items three inches away from the tip of your nose for about 30 seconds. You should guess all the items correctly. If you are successful in guessing a minimum of 5-6 items then it means that your sense of smell is above average. However, one should aim to develop 100% sense of smell.

Test II: The Family Scent Test

Pick nine essential oils viz. three from the floral family, three from spicy family and three from green family. Mix them up and smell them randomly. You can smell them with your eyes closed for better concentration. This test will enable you to find out which aroma category you like the most. Maybe, you like the floral smells better than the scent of the oil from the green family.

An aromatherapist should at least stock 30-40 types of oils. It is advisable to go in for the aromas you are naturally attracted to rather than all the essential oils that are available in the market.

The Best Essential Oils

Almost all the useful oils mix well with many other oils. Their combination have the broadest range of therapeutic uses, in addition to the most pleasant fragrance.

One can start by using a mixture of two or three or all of the following essential oils.

To begin use Lavender, Neroli, Peppermint, Sandalwood, Rose and one can add to them Eucalyptus, Geranium, Lemon, Patchouli, Chamomile, Ylang Ylang.

The five fragrance categories are:

Green

Basil	Chamomile
Clary Sage	Eucalyptus
Galbanum	Rosemary
Peppermint	Thyme
Pine	

Floral

Lavender	Neroli

Geranium   Ylang Ylang
Rose

Citrus

Lemon   Bergamot
Lemon-grass   Petitgrain
Orange

Woody

Cedarwood   Patchouli
Frankincense   Sandalwood

Spicy

Camphor   Ginger
Fennel   Juniper
Marjoram   Tea-tree
Tarragon

Mixing of Aroma Oils

Basil can be mixed with

Bergamot   Tea-tree
Cypress   Peppermint
Eucalyptus   Petitgrain
Frankincense   Pine
Geranium   Rosemary
Ginger   Clary Sage
Juniper   Tarragon
Lavender   Thyme
Lemon   Ylang Ylang
Lemon-grass

45

Bergamot can be mixed with

Basil	Cypress
Cedarwood	Fennel
Chamomile	Geranium
Ginger	Petitgrain
Juniper	Pine
Lavender	Rose
Lemon	Rosemary
Lemon-grass	Clary Sage
Marjoram	Sandalwood
Neroli	Tea-tree
Orange	Thyme
Patchouli	Ylang Ylang
Peppermint	

Camphor can be mixed with

Cedarwood	Pine
Cypress	Rosemary
Frankincense	Tarragon
Ginger	Tea-tree
Peppermint	

Cedarwood can be mixed with

Bergamot	Lavender
Camphor	Lemon
Chamomile	Neroli
Cypress	Orange
Eucalyptus	Peppermint

Fennel

Frankincense

Geranium

Juniper

Pine

Rosemary

Clary Sage

Cypress can be mixed with

Basil

Bergamot

Camphor

Cedarwood

Chamomile

Eucalyptus

Fennel

Rose

Rosemary

Frankincense

Geranium

Juniper

Lavender

Lemon

Patchouli

Pine

Clary Sage

Sandalwood

Eucalyptus can be mixed with

Basil

Cedarwood

Chamomile

Cypress

Fennel

Frankincense

Geranium

Ginger

Juniper

Lavender

Lemon

Marjoram

Peppermint

Thyme

Pine

Rosemary

Clary Sage

Sandalwood

Tea-tree

Fennel can be mixed with

Bergamot
Cedarwood
Chamomile
Cypress
Juniper
Lavender
Lemon
Peppermint
Eucalyptus
Frankincense
Geranium
Ginger
Rose
Rosemary
Sandalwood

Frankincense can be mixed with

Basil
Camphor
Cedarwood
Chamomile
Cypress
Eucalyptus
Frankincense
Fennel
Geranium
Ginger
Juniper
Lavender
Lemon
Neroli
Patchouli
Pine
Rose
Rosemary

Geranium can be mixed with

Basil
Bergamot
Cedarwood
Frankincense
Fennel
Juniper
Chamomile
Cypress
Eucalyptus
Lemon-grass
Clary Sage
Sandalwood

Lavender Ylang Ylang
Lemon

Ginger can be mixed with

Basil	Orange
Bergamot	Patchouli
Camphor	Rose
Eucalyptus	Rosemary
Frankincense	Clary Sage
Fennel	Sandalwood
Neroli	Ylang Ylang

Juniper can be mixed with

Basil	Cypress
Bergamot	Eucalyptus
Cedarwood	Fennel
Chamomile	Frankincense
Geranium	Rose
Lavender	Rosemary
Lemon	Clary Sage
Neroli	Sandalwood
Peppermint	Ylang Ylang
Petitgrain	

Lavender can be mixed with

Basil	Lemon-grass
Bergamot	Marjoram
Cedarwood	Peppermint
Chamomile	Petitgrain

Cypress	Pine
Eucalyptus	Rosemary
Fennel	Clary Sage
Frankincense	Sandalwood
Geranium	Tarragon
Juniper	Tea-tree
Lemon	Thyme

Lemon can be mixed with

Basil	Neroli
Bergamot	Orange
Cedarwood	Petitgrain
Chamomile	Pine
Cypress	Patchouli
Eucalyptus	Rose
Fennel	Rosemary
Frankincense	Sandalwood
Geranium	Tea-tree
Lavender	Ylang Ylang
Marjoram	

Marjoram can be mixed with

Basil	Juniper
Bergamot	Lavender
Chamomile	Lemon
Eucalyptus	Lemon-grass
Geranium	Neroli
Ginger	Rose

Rosemary	Sandalwood
Clary Sage	Ylang Ylang

Neroli can be mixed with

Bergamot	Marjoram
Cedarwood	Orange
Chamomile	Patchouli
Geranium	Rose
Ginger	Rosemary
Juniper	Sandalwood
Lavender	Ylang Ylang
Lemon	

Orange can be mixed with

Bergamot	Lemon
Cedarwood	Lemon-grass
Frankincense	Neroli
Geranium	Patchouli
Ginger	Petitgrain
Lavender	Pine
Rosemary	Sandalwood
Clary Sage	

Patchouli can be mixed with

Bergamot	Orange
Chamomile	Peppermint
Cypress	Pine
Frankincense	Rose
Ginger	Clary Sage

Lavender   Sandalwood
Lemon   Ylang Ylang
Marjoram

Peppermint can mixed with

Basil   Fennel
Bergamot   Juniper
Camphor   Lemon
Cedarwood   Lavender
Eucalyptus   Patchouli
Rose   Clary Sage
Rosemary   Sandalwood

Petitgrain can be mixed with

Basil   Orange
Bergamot   Rosemary
Lavender   Sandalwood
Lemon   Ylang Ylang

Pine can be mixed with

Basil   Lavender
Camphor   Lemon
Cedarwood   Orange
Chamomile   Patchouli
Cypress   Rosemary
Eucalyptus   Tea-tree
Frankincense

Rose can be mixed with

Bergamot	Cypress
Chamomile	Frankincense
Fennel	Neroli
Geranium	Patchouli
Ginger	Peppermint
Juniper	Clary Sage
Lavender	Sandalwood
Lemon	Thyme
Marjoram	

Rosemary can be mixed with

Basil	Lavender
Bergamot	Lemon
Cedarwood	Lemon-grass
Camphor	Marjoram
Chamomile	Neroli
Cypress	Orange
Eucalyptus	Peppermint
Fennel	Pine
Frankincense	Patchouli
Geranium	Sandalwood
Juniper	Thyme

Clary Sage can be mixed with

Basil	Lemon
Bergamot	Lemon-grass
Cedarwood	Marjoram

Cypress
Eucalyptus
Frankincense
Geranium
Ginger
Juniper
Lavender

Orange
Patchouli
Peppermint
Rose
Sandalwood
Ylang Ylang

Sandalwood can be mixed with

Bergamot
Cypress
Chamomile
Eucalyptus
Frankincense
Fennel
Geranium
Patchouli
Peppermint
Rose
Rosemary

Ginger
Juniper
Lavender
Lavender
Marjoram
Neroli
Orange
Clary Sage

Ylang Ylang

Tea-Tree can be mixed with

Bergamot
Chamomile
Cypress
Eucalyptus
Frankincense
Fennel
Geranium

Ginger
Juniper
Lavender
Lemon
Pine
Sandalwood

Tarragon can be mixed with

Basil	Cedarwood
Camphor	Lemongrass

Thyme can be mixed with

Basil	Chamomile
Bergamot	Eucalyptus
Lavender	Rosemary
Lemon	Clary Sage

Ylang Ylang can be mixed with

Basil	Neroli
Bergamot	Patchouli
Frankincense	Petitgrain
Geranium	Pine
Ginger	Rose
Juniper	Clary Sage
Lavender	Sandalwood
Lemon	Thyme
Marjoram	

Aroma Oils for Common Problems

Aroma oils are either relaxing, calming, stimulating or have therapeutic qualities. While using the essential oils care should be taken to dilute the oils before application.

Acne
Oils: Bergamot, Cedarwood, Geranium, Lavender, Juniper, Sandalwood, Lemon, Tea-tree, Chamomile, Petitgrain, Patchouli and Lemon-grass.

Anxiety and Stress
Oils: Lavender, Neroli, Patchouli, Sandalwood, Bergamot, Frankincense, Clary Sage and Ylang Ylang.

Athlete's Foot
Oils: Lavender, Tea-tree, Geranium and Lemon-grass.

Arthritis
Oils: Eucalyptus, Ginger, Juniper, Pine, Peppermint, Cypress, Rosemary and Lemon.

Backache
Oils: Camphor, Eucalyptus, Pine, Juniper, Petitgrain, Rosemary, Lavender, Clary Sage and Thyme.

Bites and Stings
Oils: Basil, Chamomile, Lavender, Peppermint and Tea-tree.

Breathing Problems
Oils: Cedarwood, Eucalyptus, Peppermint, Pine, Rosemary, Sandalwood and Tea-tree.

Bunion
Bunion is a painful inflammation of the joint between the big toe and the foot which is sometimes caused due to ill-fitting shoes
Oils: Cypress, Lemon and Peppermint.

Bruises
Oils: Camphor, Clary Sage, Cypress, Geranium and Lavender.

Burns
Oils: Chamomile, Geranium, Lavender, Rose and Tea-tree.

Cellulite
Cellulite (common in women) is a lumpy, dimpled, orange-peel like appearance on thighs, bottom and back of arms. It is usually caused due to accumulation of fluid and toxins in the tissues because of lack of proper circulation and due to hormonal fluctuations. Regular massage with aroma oils can help to smoothen the lumps.

Oils: Cedarwood, Clary Sage, Cypress, Geranium, Fennel, Juniper, Lemon, Lavender and Patchouli.

Chickenpox
Oils: Bergamot, Chamomile, Eucalyptus, Lavender and Tea-tree.

Chilblains
Chilblains is seen as discoloured, swollen veins on the fingers, toes and the back of legs after exposure to extremely cold weather.
Oils: Cypress, Eucalyptus, Ginger, Juniper, Lemon, Lemon-grass, Marjoram, Rosemary and Tea-tree.

Circulation (poor)
Oils: Basil, Cypress, Cedarwood, Clary Sage, Ginger, Juniper, Lemon, Lemon-grass, Lavender, Peppermint, Pine, Rosemary and Ylang Ylang.

Cold
Oils: Camphor, Eucalyptus, Lavender, Lemon, Marjoram, Peppermint, Pine, Tea-tree and Thyme.

Cough
Oils: Cedarwood, Cypress, Eucalyptus, Frankincense, Ginger, Lemon, Pine, Peppermint, Rosemary, Sandalwood and Thyme.

Cramps
Oils: Chamomile, Eucalyptus, Fennel, Juniper, Lemon, Lavender, Marjoram, Neroli, Tarragon and Ylang Ylang.

Cuts and Abrasions
Oils: Bergamot, Chamomile, Geranium, Lavender and Tea-tree.

Dandruff
Oils: Cedarwood, Geranium, Juniper, Lemon, Lavender, Rosemary, Sandalwood and Tea-tree.

Depression
Oils: Bergamot, Geranium, Clary Sage, Sandalwood, Rose, Frankincense, Neroli and Lavender, Ylang Ylang.

Dermatitis, Psoriasis, Eczema
Oils: Bergamot, Cedarwood, Chamomile, Geranium, Lavender, Sandalwood and Cypress.

Fatigue
Oils: Basil, Bergamot, Geranium, Frankincense, Eucalyptus, Lavender, Lemon, Peppermint, Clary Sage, Thyme, Ginger, Patchouli, Fennel and Orange.

Fluid Retention
Oils: Geranium, Fennel, Patchouli, Cypress, Juniper and Rosemary.

Fungal Infection
Oils: Lavender, Tea-tree, Geranium, Lemon-grass, Juniper and Sandalwood.

Hair Loss
Oils: Rosemary, Lavender, Clary Sage, Cedarwood and Ylang Ylang.

Hair (oily)
Oils: Rosemary, Lavender, Cypress, Geranium, Lemon and Tea-tree.

Hair (dry)
Oils: Chamomile for blonde hair, Rosemary, Lavender for red, brown hair and Tea-tree for dandruff.

Hangover
Oils: Geranium, Lavender, Rose, Neroli, Lemon and Peppermint.

Headache
Oils: Eucalyptus, Frankincense, Chamomile, Peppermint, Clary Sage, Lavender, Rose, Lemon-grass and Thyme.

Herpes
Oils: Bergamot, Chamomile, Eucalyptus, Lavender, Lemon, Patchouli and Tea-tree.

Household Cleansers
Oils: Geranium, Lavender Chamomile, Eucalyptus, Lemon, Tea-tree, Bergamot, Lemongrass, Thyme, Peppermint and Pine.

Indigestion
Oils: Fennel, Lavender, Peppermint, Marjoram and Tarragon.

Influenza
Oils: Eucalyptus, Peppermint, Pine, Tea-tree, Thyme, Marjoram, Orange and Rosemary.

Insomnia
Oils: Geranium, Basil, Lavender, Chamomile, Rose, Cypress, Petitgrain, Neroli, Marjoram, Sandalwood and Ylang Ylang

Insect Repellents
Oils: Camphor, Lemon-grass, Basil, Tea-tree and Thyme.

Measles
Oils: Bergamot, Eucalyptus, Chamomile, Lavender and Tea-tree.

Menopause
Oils: Chamomile, Rose, Lavender, Cypress, Geranium, Clary Sage, Peppermint and Ylang Ylang.

Nausea
Oils: Ginger, Lemon and Peppermint.

Perspiration or Excess Sweating
Oils: Bergamot, Lemon-grass, Lavender and Thyme.

Premenstrual Tension
Oils: Bergamot, Clary Sage, Cypress, Chamomile, Fennel, Geranium, Juniper, Lavender, Peppermint, Rose, Sandalwood and Tarragon.

Rheumatism
Oils: Cypress, Chamomile, Eucalyptus, Ginger, Juniper, Lavender, Lemon, Marjoram and Rosemary.

Sexual Problems
Oils: Clary Sage, Ginger, Geranium, Neroli, Patchouli, Rose, Sandalwood and Ylang Ylang.

Skin (mature)
Oils: Chamomile, Frankincense, Geranium, Lavender, Neroli, Orange, Rosemary, Rose and Ylang Ylang.

Skin (thread vein)
Oils: Chamomile, Cypress, Geranium, Orange and Lemon.

Skin (dry and sensitive)
Oils: Chamomile, Geranium, Lavender, Neroli, Patchouli, Rose, Sandalwood and Tea-tree.

Skin (oily and blemished)
Oils: Bergamot, Chamomile, Geranium, Lavender, Neroli, Cedarwood, Juniper, Lemon-grass, Petitgrain, Patchouli, Lemon and Thyme.

Stress
Oils: Basil, Bergamot, Lavender, Neroli Chamomile, Geranium, Frankincense, Clary Sage, Patchouli, Marjoram, Sandalwood and Ylang Ylang.

Sunburn
Oils: Chamomile, Geranium, Lavender and Rose.

Travel Sickness
Oils: Bergamot, Ginger, Lemon and Peppermint.

Specific Features of Aroma Oils

Analgesic (To reduce pain)
Oils: Bergamot, Chamomile, Lavender, Marjoram and Rosemary.

Antidepressant (To lift the mood)
Oils: Bergamot, Clary Sage, Chamomile, Geranium, Lavender, Neroli, Petitgrain, Rose, Orange, Sandalwood and Ylang Ylang.

Anaphrodisiac (To decrease sexual response)
Oils: Marjoram.

Anti-Inflammatory (To reduce inflammation)
Oils: Bergamot, Chamomile and Lavender.

Antiseptic (To fight bacteria locally)
Oils: Bergamot, Eucalyptus, Lavender, Juniper, Rosemary, Tea-tree and Sandalwood.

Antiviral
Oils: Tea-tree and Lavender.

Astringent
Oils: Cypress, Cedarwood, Juniper, Frankincense, Sandalwood and Rose.

Aphrodisiac (Enhance sexuality)
Oils: Rose, Neroli, Clary Sage, Sandalwood and Ylang Ylang.

Bactericide (Kills bacteria)
Oils: Bergamot, Eucalyptus, Lavender, Juniper, Rosemary and Neroli.

Cephalic (Clears the mind, stimulates mental activity)
Oils: Basil and Rosemary.

Chalagogue (To stimulate the flow of bile)
Oils: Chamomile, Lavender, Peppermint and Rosemary.

Cytophylactic (Regenerates cell)
Oils: Frankincense, Tea-tree, Lavender, Neroli and Palmarosa.

Deodorant (Reduces odour)
Oils: Clary Sage, Lavender, Neroli, Petitgrain, Eucalyptus, Lavender and Cypress.

Detoxifying (Cleanses the body of impurities)
Oils: Fennel, Juniper and Rose.

Diuretic (To increase production of urine)
Oils: Cypress, Cedarwood, Chamomile, Frankincense, Fennel, Geranium, Juniper, Rosemary and Sandalwood.

Emmenagogue (To encourage menstruation)
Oils: Basil, Clary Sage, Chamomile, Juniper, Lavender, Marjoram, Rose and Rosemary.

Expectorant (To expel phlegm)
Oils: Bergamot, Eucalyptus, Marjoram and Sandalwood.

Febrifuge (To reduce fever)
Oils: Bergamot, Chamomile, Eucalyptus, Tea-tree and Peppermint.

Fungicidal (To arrest growth of yeasts, moulds, etc)
Oils: Lavender and Tea-tree.

Hepatic (To strengthen liver)
Oils: Chamomile, Lemon, Cypress, Rosemary, Tea-tree and Lavender.

Hypertensive (To raise blood pressure)
Oils: Rosemary and Clary Sage.

Hypnotic (To induce alpha state)
Oils: Chamomile, Lavender, Neroli, Marjoram and Ylang Ylang.

Hypotensive (To lower blood pressure)
Oils: Marjoram, Lavender and Ylang Ylang.

Immunostimulant (To strengthen the body's immunity to infections)
Oils: Lavender and Tea-tree.

Nervine (To strengthen the nervous system)
Oils: Chamomile, Lavender, Marjoram and Rosemary.

Sedative (To calm the nervous system)
Oils: Bergamot, Clary Sage, Juniper, Frankincense, Lavender, Marjoram, Rose, Neroli and Sandalwood.

Stimulant (Enhances the body activity)
Oils: Black Pepper, Eucalyptus, Geranium, Rosemary and Peppermint.

Tonic (To strengthen the body generally)
Oils: Black Pepper, Basil, Chamomile, Geranium, Frankincense, Lavender, Juniper, Marjoram, Rose, Neroli and Tea-tree.

Oils to be used in moderation

Basil	Clary Sage
Camphor	Tarragon
Fennel	Thyme
Ginger	

Oils that are photo-toxic or photosensitive
Photo-toxic or photosensitivity is a reaction to essential oils causing redness, increased pigmentation and problems of the skin when in contact with the sunlight or excessive light. There is a possibility that the oils that cause photosensitivity can increase the likelihood of damage to the skin.

Bergamot	Neroli
Cedarwood	Orange (sweet and
Clary Sage	bitter)
Ginger	Patchouli
Lemon	

Oils to be avoided in pregnancy

Rosemary	Clary Sage
Basil	Cedarwood
Fennel	Juniper
Thyme	Tarragon
Marjoram	

Oils that can cause skin irritation

Basil	Lavender
Bergamot	Lemon
Black pepper	Lemon-grass
Camphor	Neroli
Cedarwood	Peppermint
Chamomile	Pine
Clove bud	Sandalwood
Eucalyptus	Tea-tree
Geranium	Thyme
Ginger	Vetiver
Juniper	Ylang Ylang

Avoid using the essential oils undiluted and insist on a skin patch test before using the aroma oils extensively on a regular basis.

Oils to be avoided while taking Homeopathic medication

The oils given below, when used while under Homeopathic medicine could neutralise the benefits of the Homeopathic remedies, therefore they should be avoided.

Black Pepper   Eucalyptus
Camphor   Peppermint
Clove bud   Rosemary

Oils to be avoided when driving (long distance)

The following oils should be avoided when driving, because these can cause drowsiness when one has to be alert.

Chamomile   Petitgrain
Geranium   Rose
Lavender   Sandalwood
Marjoram   Vetiver
Neroli   Ylang Ylang

Oils that can be contra-indicators during certain illness

Condition		Contra-indicator oil
Asthma	:	Marjoram, Camphor, Rosemary.
Anorexia	:	Patchouli.
Cancer	:	Basil, Fennel.
Epilepsy	:	Clary Sage, Fennel, Eucalyptus, Lavender, Rosemary.

Hypertension	:	Rosemary, Thyme.
Hypotension	:	Marjoram, Clary Sage.
Liver disease	:	Clove bud, Thyme, Vetiver.
Ulcers of the stomach and intestine	:	Cinnamon.

Carrier Oils

Carrier oils or base oils are vegetable, nut or seed oils. Many of these carrier oils also have therapeutic properties. Vegetable oils are extracted from the seeds of the plants. Vegetable oils contain a good amount of proteins, nutrients and energy. They enable the body to produce heat and lubrication.

The essential oils are very highly concentrated and cannot be used directly on the skin. The essential oils hence are diluted with a base or carrier oil, so that they can be massaged or rubbed into the skin in the correct proportion.

Almond Oil (Sweet)

Colour : very pale yellow.

Extracted : from the kernel.

Contains : glycosides, minerals, vitamins and proteins.

Uses : good for skin, helps relieve itching, soreness, dryness and inflammation.

Base oil : can be used as a base without dilution.

Apricot Kernel Oil

Colour	:	pale yellow.
Extracted	:	from the kernel.
Contains	:	minerals, vitamins.
Uses	:	all types of skin particularly for premature aging, sensitive, inflamed and dry skin.
Base oil	:	can be used as a base without dilution.

Avocado-Pear Oil

Colour	:	dark green.
Extracted	:	from the fruit.
Contains	:	vitamins, proteins, lecithin and fatty acids.
Uses	:	all types of skin especially dry and dehydrated skin, eczema.
Base oil	:	to be used as an addition to a base oil in 10% dilution.

Carrot Oil

Colour	:	orange.
Contains	:	vitamins, minerals, and beta-carotene.
Uses	:	premature aging, itching, dryness, psoriasis and eczema. Very rejuvenating, reduces scarring.

Base oil : to be used as an addition to a base oil in 10% dilution. Do not use undiluted oil directly on the skin.

Corn oil

Colour : pale yellow.
Contains : vitamins, minerals and protein.
Uses : soothing for all types of skin.
Base oil : can be used as base oil.

Evening Primrose

Colour : pale yellow.
Contains : gamma linolenic acid, vitamins and minerals.
Uses : during Premenstrual tension, multiple sclerosis, menopause related tensions, and heart diseases. Excellent while treating eczema and psoriasis. Helps prevent premature aging of skin.
Base oil : use with 10% dilution.

Grapeseed oil

Colour : nearly colourless or pale green.
Contains : vitamins, minerals and protein.
Uses : for all types of skin.
Base oil : can be used as base oil without dilution.

Hazelnut oil

Colour   : yellow.
Extracted   : from the kernel.
Contains   : vitamins, minerals and protein.
Uses   : for all types of skin. It has a slight astringent action.
Base oil   : use with 10% dilution.

Jojoba oil

Colour   : yellow.
Extracted   : from the bean.
Contains   : minerals, protein, a waxy substance similar to collagen.
Uses   : for inflamed skins, psoriasis, eczema, acne, hair care. It can be used on all types of skin as it is a very penetrative oil.
Base oil   : can be used as base oil without dilution.

Olive oil

Colour   : green.
Contains   : vitamins, minerals, protein.
Uses   : rheumatism, hair care, cosmetics. It is a very soothing oil.
Base oil   : use with 10% dilution.

Peanut oil

Colour	:	pale yellow.
Contains	:	vitamins, minerals and protein.
Uses	:	for all types of skin.
Base oil	:	can be used as base oil without dilution.

Safflower oil

Colour	:	pale yellow.
Contains	:	vitamins, minerals and protein.
Uses	:	for all types of skin.
Base oil	:	can be used as base oil without dilution.

Sesame oil

Colour	:	dark yellow.
Contains	:	vitamins, minerals, protein, lecithin and amino acids.
Uses	:	rheumatism, arthritis, psoriasis, eczema. Useful for all skin types.
Base oil	:	use in 10% dilution.

Soya bean oil

Colour	:	pale yellow.
Contains	:	vitamins, minerals and protein.
Uses	:	for all types of skin.
Base oil	:	can be used as base oil without dilution.

Sunflower oil

Colour	:	pale yellow.
Contains	:	vitamins and minerals.
Uses	:	for all types of skin.
Base oil	:	can be used as base oil without dilution.

Equipment Required for Mixing Oils

After studying the feature, properties or category, select the essential oils you wish to mix and use. It is preferable not to mix more than three oils at a time. Also select the oils belonging to the same category. For example if you want to use more than one oil select them all from either floral, spicy, citrus, green or woody. Hence you could try out a mixture of perhaps lavender, rose and ylang ylang as all these belong to the floral family.

Once you have selected the oils that you want to mix and use, try the combination in a smaller quantity before you mix a large quantity so as to not waste the oils. Cut long strips of blotting paper, put a drop of each of the selected oils in case you wish to use equal amounts of all the oils selected. In case you have decided to use any one or two of the selected oil more than the other, add two drops of those. Now hold the strip and move the oily tip of the blotting paper backward and forward under your nose as you inhale the aroma. Allow your sense of smell to be the judge and guide you in selecting the combinations.

Since aromatherapy is very personal you should get the other person to do a similar test before mixing a combination because it is not necessary that the mixture selected by you and liked by you should necessarily be liked by others too.

Equipment

- 10 ml. dark coloured glass bottles with stoppered caps for storing pure essential oils.
- Four eye-droppers or pipettes. You could use one only if you thoroughly wash it every time after use.
- A small funnel for pouring carrier oils into bottles.
- A large, dark coloured glass, stoppered bottles for storing the combinations of oils or a ceramic bowl for immediate use. Please do not use metal containers or bowls.
- Strips of blotting paper.

How to Select Essential Oils?

The Best Aroma Oils:

Clary Sage	Peppermint
Eucalyptus	Petitgrain
Geranium	Rosemary
Lavender	Tea-tree
Lemon	Ylang Ylang

Male Favourites:

Basil	Lemon
Bergamot	Patchouli
Eucalyptus	Pine
Frankincense	Sandalwood
Lavender	

Female Favourites:

Bergamot	Lavender
Geranium	Neroli
Patchouli	Clary Sage
Peppermint	Ylang Ylang
Rose	

Caution to be Exercised
While Using Aroma Oils

Skin Patch Test

To test aroma oil blended with carrier or base oils

- Wash and dry the forearm thoroughly.
- Apply just a few drops of the blended aroma oil to moisten the area.
- Cover the area with a sterile gauze.
- Let it remain for 24 hours.
- If there is irritation then wash immediately.
- In case of irritation, you should not use this oil.

To test essential oil in its pure state

- Wash and dry the forearm thoroughly with an unscented vegetable soap.
- Apply one drop of the aroma oil to the crook of the arm.
- Bend the arm so that it touches the shoulder for five minutes.
- Open and close once more.

If any irritation occurs wash immediately with water and soap or wipe carefully with a cotton ball soaked in milk and vegetable oil.

Aroma oils being potent, safety precautions need to be followed with utmost care. Do not allow children to play with these oils and always store them away from the reach of children and other non-qualified users of essential oils.

In case accidental poisoning occurs follow the following :

In Eyes

In case essential oil comes in contact with the eyes, do not rinse with water. But instead wipe the eye with a ball of cotton soaked in milk or vegetable oil. If irritation still persists wash the eyes with water poured from a jug, from a height of 3-5 inches for 15 minutes. Consult a doctor. It always helps to wash the eyes for 10 to 15 minutes than splashing it with running water.

Toxic Effects

When the oil is not evenly spread out on the area and remains concentrated in one area in a large quantity it can have a toxic effect. Even daily exposure to the same oil on a regular basis for a prolonged period can lead to toxicity. Symptoms that would follow a toxic reaction are fatigue, headaches, liver pain, liver enlargement, coughing and urine disturbances. This make it mandatory for the therapists using essential oils to work in a well ventilated room and wash their hands thoroughly after handling the oils.

Allergic Effects

An allergic reaction to aroma oil would result in nausea, dizziness, sweating, stomachache, irritation of the mucous membrane and palpitation. These allergic reactions are temporary and would cease to exist as soon as the use of the essential oils is stopped.

The toxicity of the essential oils depends on the level of toxicity and concentration of the chemical compounds. All aroma oils need to be used as per instructions only and more so when handling those essential oils under toxic listing. Normally, a toxic reaction occurs when the essential oil is used in excess or incorrectly. It is safer to use the aroma oils under proper guidance and instructions.

The following precautions needs to be followed while dealing with essential oils having toxic rating:

- Do not exceed the recommended dosage.
- If you feel uncomfortable even while using the recommended dosage reduce the dosage to half.
- Follow the skin patch test carefully.
- Avoid usage for a long period. The maximum administration time should not exceed 2 – 4 weeks. Leave a gap of 30 days before beginning to use again.

- Avoid use during pregnancy.
- Do not use if you are a nursing mother.
- Do not administer on infants, small children, frail or elderly people who have less resistance.

Different Ways of Using Essential Oils

Method and Usage

Rub oil : 8-10 drops of essential oil in 10ml. base oil. Use only 4-6 drops once a day, preferably at night

Baths : 6-8 drops in a tub, 2-3 drops in a bucket once a day

Shower : 10-12 drops in 10 ml. base oil once a day. Wash as usual. Add oil on your face towel, cloth or sponge or use your hands and rub briskly all over the body as you stand under the running shower. Breathe deeply to benefit from the aromatic vapour.

Massage oil : 8-10 drops of essential oil for every 30 ml. of vegetable base oil once a day

Diffuser : 1-6 drops

Inhalation	:	2-3 drops once a day
	:	1-2 drops on a tissue. Sniff when required. Keep the tissue under the pillow during the night
	:	2-3 drops of essential oil on a piece of cotton and left for 10-15 minutes to dry. This piece of cotton can be kept in the cupboard, car, shoe rack, lockers etc.
Water bowls	:	1-9 drops of aroma oil to be added to bowl of boiling water. Keep in the room and close the windows, door and allow the aroma to spread in the room. This can also be used in work places.
Room sprays	:	4-6 drops can be added to 30 ml. of water in a spray bottle. Shake well and spray the mixture in the air. Avoid spraying directly on delicate machines. Ideal for home and office use.

Careful Handling of the Essential Oils

- Essential oils are not recommended for internal consumption.
- Certain oils are to be avoided during early pregnancy as they can induce menstruation and some even have diuretic properties which can deplete the fluid in the foetal sack. These oils include Basil, Clary Sage, Rosemary, Juniper, Marjoram, Clove bud, Fennel, Cypress, Peppermint, Cedarwood. However, this caution does not apply to oils used in vaporisers.
- Avoid exposure to sun for at least four hours after using essential oils as some oils can make the skin photosensitive to ultraviolet rays from the sun. Bergamot, Lemon, Orange, Petitgrain are some such oils that can cause photosensitivity.
- People suffering from high blood pressure, epilepsy, neural disorders or kidney disease should avoid some oils viz. Black Pepper, Rosemary, Cypress, Juniper.

- Aroma oils are not a substitute for any drugs being taken under the advice of a qualified physician for serious ailments. It is always advisable to consult a qualified therapist before considering the use of essential oils particularly when suffering from serious ailments.

- Use the oils in recommended dosage. Usage in excess can lead to opposite effect to that which you are trying to achieve and there are chances of building up of the toxicity within the body. Ylang Ylang, marjoram, Clary Sage need to be used with utmost precaution.

- Essential oils should always be used after dilution unless recommended otherwise.

- Keep out of reach of children.

- Store the oils only in dark glass containers. The colour of the bottle should preferably be amber rather than cobalt blue. Only blended oils should be stored in cobalt blue bottles.

- Store in a cool, dark place away from sunlight to prolong the life of the aroma oils and also to preserve the therapeutic powers of the essential oils.

- Avoid using essential oils near the eyes or other sensitive areas.

- Avoid contact with plastic, varnished or painted surfaces.

- When blending essential oils use a stainless steel, glass or ceramic container and not plastic.
- Do not use essential oils on newborn. Use only one drop of lavender in the bath until the age of four months. For the use of essential oils on children up to the age of 12 years, a quarter of a dosage given to an adult should be utilized.
- What suits one may not necessarily suit another person.
- Avoid certain aroma oils under the influence of alcohol. Oils viz. Clary Sage, Marjoram, Ylang Ylang should particularly be avoided in case alcohol has been taken.
- Some oils may irritate the skin. Always do a skin patch test before applying the oils to larger area.
- If you are not sure of a particular blend, it is always better to take advise from a professional aromatherapist.

How Aroma Oils Are Made?

Distillation

Water distillation for dried material that will not get damaged by boiling. This method is also used for powdered materials and flowers like rose and orange flowers

Water and Steam distillation for dried and fresh material that would get damaged by boiling. In this method they are supported on a perforated grid and steam is passed through them like cinnamon and clove.

Direct steam distillation for fresh plant material having a high boiling point, steam is passed at a high temperature (seeds, roots, wood). Also applicable for fresh plant material like peppermint.

Cold pressing or extraction

It is mainly for citrus oils like lemon and orange. The fruit is rolled over sharp projections that puncture the oil glands. Fruit is then pressed to remove the oil and then washed off with a fine spray of water. Rotating the mixture at a very high speed separates oil and water. The fruit can also first be separated from the peel and then cold pressed like bergamot.

Carbon dioxide extraction

Liquid CO_2 is used as a solvent to extract essential oils. Liquefied under pressure, it acts as a solvent, reverting back to gaseous nature when pressure is reduced leaving no trace of the solvent.

Solvent extraction

Volatile solvents like petroleum, ether, benzene or hexane are mixed into petals till the essential oil is completely dissolved. Filtration is followed by reduced pressure and evaporation of the solvent to give concrete products which contains insoluble vegetable wax or pigments. On continuing the process with solvents and freezing it finally separates the waxes and gives the final product which is called absolute.

Aroma Oil and Beauty Care

Suggested blends for skin types

Normal skin : Lavender, Geranium, Rosemary, Cedarwood, Orange.

Dry skin : Lavender, Geranium, Cedarwood, Patchouli, Frankincense, Sandalwood, Ylang Ylang.

Oily skin : Cedarwood, Lavender, Rosemary, Frankincense, Orange, Cypress, Bergamot, Juniper, Lemon-grass, Clary Sage, Lemon.

Mature skin : Frankincense, Sandalwood, Ylang Ylang, Patchouli, Cypress, Lavender, Geranium.

Blemished skin : Lavender, Geranium, Rosemary, Lemon, Tea-tree.

Sensitive skin : Lavender, Sandalwood, Cedarwood.

Moisturisers

Add the following blends to 50 ml. of unscented moisturiser base:

Day Cream (Dry Skin)

2 drops of Wheat Germ
4 drops of Lavender
2 drops of Ylang Ylang
4 drops of Frankincense

Night Cream (Dry Skin)

1 ml. Jojoba
6 drops of Geranium
4 drops of Sandalwood
2 drops of Frankincense

Pimple Ointment

8 drops of Lavender
1 drop of Peppermint
4 drops of Tea-tree

Day Cream (Oily Skin)

2 drops of Wheat Germ
2 drops of Lemon
3 drops of Lavender
2 drops of Cypress
2 drops of Juniper

Hair care

Suggested oils for hair types

Dry hair   :   Rosemary, Sandalwood, Ylang
                     Ylang, Lavender, Geranium,
                     Frankincense, Patchouli.

Oily hair	:	Basil, Eucalyptus, Cedarwood, Lemon-grass, Cypress, Rosemary, Bergamot, Juniper.
Normal hair	:	Geranium, Lemon, Lemongrass, Clary Sage, Cedarwood, Rosemary.
Dandruff	:	Cedarwood, Eucalyptus, Clary Sage, Patchouli, Rosemary, Tea-Tree, Lavender.
Brittled or Damaged	:	Sandalwood, Geranium, Lavender, Frankincense, Patchouli.

A special scalp treatment for brittle or damaged hair:
Take 10 ml. Jojoba
Five drops of dry hair type combination
Method: Warm the blends in a dish. Massage the mixture into the scalp. Saturate some cotton wool and rub through to the ends of the hair. Wrap a hot towel around your head. Leave for 15 minutes and then shampoo.

Treat Your Feet

Tired feet :
2 drops of Orange
3 drops of Rosemary
3 drops of Lavender

Smelly feet
3 drops of Cypress
3 drops of Lemon-grass
2 drops of Tea-tree

Swollen feet
3 drops of Juniper
3 drops of Lavender
2 drops of Peppermint

Feet Energiser
3 drops of Bergamot
3 drops of Clary Sage
2 drops of Juniper

With the above combination you can enjoy a 15-minute aromatic foot bath at any time of day. These can also be blended and diluted in 20 ml. carrier oils to make a refreshing foot massage.

Treat Your Hands

Normal skin
2 drops of Lavender
2 drops of Geranium
3 drops of Sandalwood

Dry skin
2 drops of Lavender
2 drops of Frankincense
2 drops of Patchouli

Arthritic hands

3 drops of Juniper

2 drops or Rosemary

1 drop of Cypress

Add any of the above in 15 ml. carrier oil and massage into the hands including the forearm. Before the massage soak hands in warm water in which you have dropped three drops of Lavender to soften the skin.

How to Use Aroma Oils?

All the above oils are ready to use and are mixed with carefully selected carrier oils. They can be used in two ways.

- Rub on the skin locally as required and allow the oil to be absorbed into the blood stream because the oil molecules are so small that they can be absorbed through the pores of the skin or add the aroma oil to the massage oil to obtain higher benefits for the whole body following this by steam or sauna could be a rejuvenating and refreshing feeling.

- Direct inhalation or steam inhalation; sprinkle one or two drops of the chosen oil on a handkerchief and inhale the oil while at work or travelling. A couple of drops of relaxing oil on a tissue inside your pillow helps you to sleep peacefully. Steam inhalations with two drops of aroma oil in a bowl of hot water also helps. You can also use it in the bath water (in bathtub about 6-8 drops, in bucket 2-3 drops) wraps, compress, massage, inhalation and diffusers. It is advisable to do a patch test before use of any essential oil. Apply at the back of the elbow or wrist and leave for 24 hour without washing the area. If there is no allergy you can comfortably use the oil. Avoid contact with plastic, varnished or painted surfaces. Avoid sensitive areas and eyes. Wash hands after handling the oil. Do not use while taking homeopathic treatment or internal consumption. Do not use for babies. Aroma oils are not a substitute for any drugs that are being taken. They can be a complementary therapy. Pregnant ladies and individuals suffering from blood pressure, heart ailment, epilepsy are requested to consult qualified therapists before using essential oils.